STAPH INFECTIONS

PRACTICAL GUIDE TO DEALING WITH

STAPH INFECTIONS

DR. J. WALLER

Contents

INTRODUCTION 3

CHAPTER ONE 6

What Staph Infections Are 6

Staph Infection Types.......................................10

Reasons and Danger Elements.......................15

CHAPTER TWO 16

Signs and symptoms..21

Identification and Medical Assessment 26

Methods of Therapy..31

CHAPTER THREE 37

Preventive Actions 37

Issues and Prolonged Effects 43

CONCLUSION...48

THE END 51

INTRODUCTION

The Staphylococcus genus of bacteria is the source of staph infections, a category of infections that can range in severity from minor skin ailments to serious and often fatal disorders. Human skin and mucous membranes are frequently home to Staphylococcus bacteria, which, although generally coexisting innocuously, can cause infections when they penetrate the body through cuts, wounds, or other openings.

One of the main characteristics of staph infections is their capacity to cause a broad spectrum of symptoms and impact different body areas. The kind of Staphylococcus bacteria involved, the person's general health, and the immune system's reaction all affect how serious the infection is.

One prevalent species of Staphylococcus that can infect people is Staphylococcus aureus. Methicillin-resistant Staphylococcus aureus (MRSA) is a difficult-to-treat form of bacteria that has acquired resistance to several medications.

Skin infections like cellulitis, impetigo, and boils are common kinds of Staph infections. In addition to respiratory infections and food poisoning, Staph bacteria can also cause more serious illnesses like pneumonia and bloodstream infections.

Depending on the type and location of the infection, diagnosis of Staph infections usually entails a clinical examination, laboratory testing, and occasionally imaging techniques. Antibiotics may be used in treatment, but the exact strain of Staphylococcus and how susceptible it is to them will determine which drug is best.

Keeping wounds clean and covered, washing your hands frequently, maintaining proper hygiene, and avoiding contact with contaminated surfaces or infected people are all examples of preventive actions. Comprehending the indications and obtaining immediate medical assistance are essential for effectively managing Staph infections.

CHAPTER ONE

What Staph Infections Are

Staphylococcal infections, or staph infections for short, are bacterial infections brought on by different Staphylococcus species. The most prevalent and clinically significant species linked to infections in humans is Staphylococcus aureus. Although these bacteria are normally harmless when present on the skin and mucous membranes, when they go inside the body through cuts, wounds, or other holes, they can cause infections.

Important Points:

Gram-positive, spherical Staphylococcus bacteria are frequently found on the skin, in the nose, and on other mucous membranes.

Staph infections are frequently opportunistic diseases, meaning they take advantage of skin holes or compromised immune systems to spread.

Severity Range: Staph infections can range in severity from less serious skin ailments like impetigo or boils to more serious and potentially fatal infections that damage internal organs and systems.

Resistant Strains: Methicillin-resistant Staphylococcus aureus (MRSA) is a strain that is difficult to treat because it has become resistant to several drugs.

Frequently Infected Sites:

Skin infections include cellulitis, impetigo, and boils.

Pneumonia is a respiratory infection.

Food Poisoning: Toxins generated by bacteria that induce food poisoning due to Staphylococcus bacterium.

Symptoms: These might include redness, swelling, soreness, fever, and in more serious cases, systemic symptoms. Symptoms can vary depending on the type and location of the infection.

Diagnosis: To ascertain the kind and severity of the illness, the diagnosis process includes a clinical examination, laboratory testing (such as cultures), and occasionally imaging scans.

Treatment: Antibiotics are the usual course of treatment; however, the particular strain and its antibiotic susceptibility will determine the drug to be used. Infected fluids or abscesses may also need to be drained.

Prevention: Keeping wounds clean, avoiding contact with infected people, using the proper antibiotics under medical supervision, and practicing excellent hygiene are all examples of preventive strategies.

Because Staph bacteria are resistant to many medications, particularly MRSA, infections can be difficult to treat. Accurate diagnosis, suitable therapy, and prophylactic actions are critical to controlling and reducing the consequences of Staph infections.

Staph Infection Types

Staph infections can affect different sections of the body and take on different shapes. Staph infections can range in severity from minor cutaneous diseases to serious systemic infections that could be fatal. The following are a few typical Staph infection types:

Skin infections:

Boils: Infected hair follicles cause painful, pus-filled lumps to develop beneath the skin.

Impetigo: A communicable skin infection marked by blisters that form from red lesions that may leak liquid.

Cellulitis: An infection that results in redness, swelling, and pain in the skin's deeper layers.

Infections of Soft Tissue:

Abscesses: A buildup of pus inside tissues that frequently need to be drained in order to be treated.

Inflammation of the hair follicles that results in pustules or red lumps is known as foliculitis.

infected respiratory systems:

Pneumonia: Respiratory symptoms and lung inflammation can result from Staphylococcus aureus-caused pneumonia.

Foodborne Illness:

Food poisoning caused by Staphylococcus aureus toxins is known as staphylococcal food poisoning. Nausea, vomiting, cramping in the abdomen, and diarrhea are some of the symptoms.

infections of the bloodstream:

Staphylococcus bacteria in the circulation, known as "bacteremia," can cause sepsis if left untreated.

infected bones and joints:

Osteomyelitis: Bone infection, usually following an accident or skin infection.

Septic arthritis is a joint infection that results in pain, edema, and restricted movement.

Infections of the heart valves:

An infection of the inner lining of the heart's chambers and valves is known as infectious endocarditis.

Syndrome of Toxic Shock (TSS):

a rare yet dangerous illness that manifests as a sudden high temperature, rash, hypotension, and multiple organ failure.

Hospital-Area Infections:

surgical site infections, especially following surgeries involving implants or prosthetic devices.

Infernal Fasciitis:

a serious soft tissue infection that is spreading quickly, has the potential to kill tissue, and needs to be treated very once.

Infections of the eyes:

It is possible to develop staphylococcal conjunctivitis or eye infections, which can hurt and cause redness and discharge.

It is noteworthy that antibiotic resistance in Staph infections, particularly those resulting from methicillin-resistant Staphylococcus aureus (MRSA), may necessitate particular treatment strategies. Effective management of Staph infections requires timely medical attention, accurate diagnosis, and focused therapy.

Reasons and Danger Elements

Staphylococcus aureus is the most frequent cause of staph infections, which are caused by bacteria belonging to the Staphylococcus genus. These bacteria can cause infections when they penetrate the body through skin cracks or other openings. They are typically found on the skin and mucous membranes. The causes and risk factors of Staph infections are influenced by multiple variables:

CHAPTER TWO

1. Breaks in the Skin:

Abrasions, cuts, wounds, and surgical incisions are all potential entrance sites for the Staphylococcus bacteria. Additionally, skin-to-skin contact can aid in transmission.

2. Reduced Immune Response:

Staph infections are more common in people with compromised immune systems, such as those with HIV/AIDS, cancer, or taking immunosuppressive therapy.

3. Long-Term Medical Conditions:

Chronic illnesses such as diabetes, heart disease, or lung disease can make it more difficult for the body to fight off infections.

4. Hospital or Medical Facilities:

Hospitals and healthcare facilities are more likely to experience healthcare-associated Staph infections, particularly those brought on by methicillin-resistant Staphylococcus aureus (MRSA).

5. Medical Procedures That Intrude:

Staph bacteria can enter the body through invasive procedures, surgeries, or the use of medical devices (implants, catheters).

6. Skin Issues:

Staph infections can arise from skin disorders like dermatitis or eczema that produce breaches in the skin.

7. Tight or Congested Living Spaces:

Close-knit environments like jails, military barracks, or densely populated homes raise the possibility of person-to-person transmission.

8. Bad Personal Hygiene Habits:

Inadequate hand hygiene has the potential to spread Staph infections, particularly in medical environments and among people who have poor personal hygiene.

9. Exchanging Individual Goods:

People who share personal goods such as towels, razors, or sports equipment might spread Staph bacteria to one another.

10. Age:

Due to their growing or compromised immune systems, infants and the elderly may be more vulnerable to Staph infections.

11. Use of Intravenous Drugs:

The risk of bloodstream infections and Staphylococcus aureus-related problems is increased with intravenous drug usage.

12. Social Environments:

Staph infections linked to the community, such as skin and soft tissue infections, can strike otherwise healthy people.

13. Past Staph Incidents:

People with a history of Staph infections, particularly those that are difficult to cure or recurrent, may be more susceptible.

14. Use of Antibiotics:

The balance of microorganisms on the skin and mucous membranes can be upset by prolonged or improper use of antibiotics, which may encourage Staph infections.

It is essential to comprehend these causes and risk factors in order to implement early intervention and preventative actions. Reducing the risk of Staph infections involves practicing excellent hygiene, leading a healthy lifestyle, and getting medical help as soon as possible for infections or skin injuries. Antibiotic stewardship and infection control practices are crucial in stopping the spread of Staphylococcus germs in healthcare environments.

Signs and symptoms

Depending on the body part afflicted, the type and intensity of the infection, and other factors, the symptoms of Staph infections can differ significantly. The following are typical signs of several Staph infection types:

1. Skin infections:

Boils: Pus-filled, red, swollen bumps that hurt.

Impetigo: Red sores that develop into blisters and may leak fluid, leaving behind a crust that looks like honey.

Cellulitis is characterized by red, puffy, and sensitive skin that frequently spreads from the site of an injury or lesion and may also be heated.

2. Infections of Soft Tissue:

Abscesses: Pupils gathered in tissues that produce discomfort, swelling, and redness.

Inflammation of the hair follicles that results in pustules or red lumps is known as foliculitis.

3. infected respiratory systems:

Chest pain, fever, shortness of breath, and cough are some of the signs of pneumonia.

4. Foodborne Illness:

Food poisoning caused by Staphylococcus bacteria: Usually manifests as diarrhea, cramping in the abdomen, vomiting, and nausea a few hours after eating tainted food.

5. infections of the bloodstream:

Bacteremia: fever, chills, hypotension, and other sepsis-related symptoms.

6. infected bones and joints:

Osteomyelitis: restricted joint motion, redness, edema, and pain in the bones.

Septic arthritis manifests as warmth, edema, pain in the joints, and limited range of motion.

7. Infections of the heart valves:

The symptoms of infectious endocarditis can include joint discomfort, weariness, fever, and heart murmurs.

8. Syndrome of Toxic Shock (TSS):

abrupt onset of diarrhea, vomiting, low blood pressure, rash, and high temperature.

9. Hospital-Area Infections:

discomfort, drainage, edema, and redness at the surgical site.

10. Infernal Fasciitis:

Excruciating pain, redness, and swelling at the infection site that quickly progresses to tissue necrosis.

11. Infections of the eyes:

The symptoms of staphylococcal conjunctivitis include ocular redness, discharge, and pain.

It is noteworthy that treating Staph infections can be increasingly difficult due to drug resistance, particularly those caused by methicillin-resistant Staphylococcus aureus (MRSA). Staph infections can sometimes spread quickly and result in life-threatening consequences, underscoring the significance of receiving treatment as soon as possible.

People who exhibit symptoms that could indicate a Staph infection should see a doctor for a proper diagnosis and course of treatment, particularly if they are accompanied by a fever or other systemic symptoms. Early action lowers the chance of complications and helps stop the infection from spreading.

Identification and Medical Assessment

A combination of clinical examination, laboratory testing, and, in certain situations, imaging techniques is usually used to diagnose and medically assess Staph infections. The following are the main facets of the medical assessment and diagnosis of Staph infections:

1. Clinical Assessment:

A medical professional will perform a comprehensive physical examination, paying close attention to the problematic area or areas. They will evaluate the presence of skin lesions, inflammatory indicators, and any accompanying symptoms.

2. Health Background:

It is imperative to compile a thorough medical history. Understanding the infection's background requires knowledge of recent injuries, operations, hospital stays, exposure to medical facilities, and the existence of underlying medical disorders.

3. Laboratory Examinations:

Gathering samples from the afflicted area, such as nasal swabs, blood, or wound drainage, for laboratory analysis is known as "culture and sensitivity testing." This aids in identifying the particular Staphylococcus strain and figuring out how sensitive it is to antibiotics.

Blood Cultures: Blood cultures can be used to find out whether there are any bacteria in the bloodstream if a bloodstream infection is suspected.

4. Imaging Research:

Imaging tests could be requested in some circumstances to determine the depth of the illness or whether deeper tissues are affected. Depending on the location and severity of the infection, various imaging modalities such as CT, MRI, ultrasound, and X-rays may be employed.

5. Molecular Examining:

Molecular testing techniques such as polymerase chain reaction (PCR) can be utilized to identify particular genes linked to antibiotic resistance, particularly in the context of methicillin-resistant Staphylococcus aureus (MRSA).

6. autopsy

The extent of tissue damage may be determined by performing a biopsy of the damaged tissue if there is a suspicion of more serious infections or consequences such necrotizing fasciitis.

7. Evaluation of Systemic Indications:

Assessing systemic symptoms, such fever, hypotension, and other sepsis-related indicators, is crucial in figuring out how serious the infection is and whether hospitalization is necessary.

8. Evaluation of the Supporting Conditions:

recognizing and treating underlying medical issues, such as diabetes or immunosuppression, that may exacerbate or prolong Staph infections.

9. Testing for Allergies:

Determining the best course of treatment requires testing for allergies and severe antibiotic reactions.

The presumed type and location of the Staph infection determine which diagnostic tests should be ordered. Timely and tailored treatment must begin with an accurate and timely diagnosis. Based on the detected strain and its antibiotic sensitivity, the proper antibiotics or other treatment modalities are administered once a diagnosis is established. Ensuring best results and avoiding problems requires careful monitoring and follow-up of the therapy response.

Methods of Therapy

The nature and intensity of the illness, along with variables like the antibiotic susceptibility of the particular strain of Staphylococcus bacteria, all influence the treatment strategies for Staph infections. These are typical methods of treatment:

1. Antibiotics:

The mainstay of care for Staph infections is antibiotics. The strain that has been identified and its medication susceptibility determine which antibiotics should be used.

Alternative antibiotics like vancomycin, daptomycin, or linezolid may be used to treat methicillin-resistant Staphylococcus aureus (MRSA).

2. Emptying Abscesses:

Pus drainage may be required for infections of the skin and soft tissues resulting in the formation of an abscess. A medical expert can accomplish this through incision and drainage.

3. Handling Injuries:

Treatment of wounds properly is crucial for skin infections. Wounds that are kept dry, clean, and covered aid in the healing process and help stop new infections.

4. Assistive Healthcare:

Pain reduction, fever control, and treating systemic symptoms related to the infection are examples of supportive interventions.

5. Bedding in:

Hospitalization may be necessary for intravenous antibiotics, intensive observation, and supportive care in cases of severe Staph infections, particularly those affecting the bloodstream, bones, or deep tissues.

6. Surgical Procedure:

Surgical intervention may be required in situations of infections affecting the bones (osteomyelitis), joints (septic arthritis), or severe soft tissues in order to drain abscesses, remove contaminated tissue, or treat sequelae.

7. Antibiotic Management:

It's critical to utilize antibiotics appropriately. In order to reduce the risk of antibiotic resistance and side effects, healthcare providers adhere to antibiotic stewardship standards.

8. Continuation Care:

It's critical to follow up with medical professionals on a regular basis to evaluate treatment response, look for any problems, and modify the treatment plan as necessary.

9. Stopping the Spread:

Infection control strategies are used in hospital settings to stop Staph infections from spreading. This entails using personal protective equipment, washing your hands properly, and keeping sick people isolated.

10. Taking Care of the Underlying Conditions

Determining and treating underlying illnesses or risk factors (such as immunosuppression or diabetes) that are causing the Staph infection.

11. A Look at Allergies:

Alternative drugs may be chosen if the patient has allergies or experiences negative reactions to specific antibiotics.

It is noteworthy that the advent of strains that are resistant to antibiotics, particularly MRSA, presents difficulties in the management of Staph infections. Testing for antibiotic susceptibility may be something that healthcare practitioners need to take into account and modify treatment strategies for.

People who experience systemic symptoms, fever, or skin lesions that could indicate a Staph infection should get medical help right away to ensure a proper diagnosis and course of treatment. For a favorable outcome and to avoid complications, early intervention is essential.

CHAPTER THREE

Good hygiene habits, infection control strategies, and lifestyle decisions that lower the chance of coming into contact with Staphylococcus bacteria are all important components of preventing Staph infections. The following are precautions against Staph infections:

1. Hand Sanitization:

Frequently wash your hands with soap and water, especially before eating, after using the restroom, and after being in a crowded or public place.

2. Suitable Closure Management:

Cuts, wounds, and skin lesions should be cleaned thoroughly and covered with sterile bandages to stop the Staph bacteria from entering the body.

3. Steer clear of skin-to-skin contact:

Reduce the amount of time that people are in direct touch with wounds, lesions, or infected regions to stop the spread of Staph bacteria.

4. Individual cleanliness:

To ensure proper personal hygiene, bathe frequently and keep your skin clean. Focus on places where perspiration and bacterial colonization are likely to occur.

5. Steer clear of shared personal items:

Towels, razors, and clothes are examples of personal goods that should not be shared as this can spread the Staph bacteria.

6. sanitizing and disinfecting:

To lower the danger of contamination, surfaces should be cleaned and disinfected on a regular basis, particularly in hospital settings.

7. Handling Food Properly:

To avoid contracting staphylococcal food poisoning, follow proper food hygiene practices, such as fully cooking meat and storing perishable goods.

8. Antibiotic Management:

Use antibiotics sparingly and only as directed by medical professionals to stop the emergence of Staphylococcus strains that are resistant to them.

9. Vaccination:

Remain up to date on your vaccinations because some of them can shield you against Staphylococcus aureus-related respiratory illnesses.

10. Hospital-related Infection Control:

To prevent Staph infections linked to healthcare, follow infection control procedures in healthcare settings, such as hand cleanliness, wearing personal protective equipment, and handling medical instruments properly.

11. Knowledge and Consciousness:

Raise awareness in community and medical settings about Staph infections and precautions to take. People who are well-informed are better equipped to lower their risk of illness.

12. A Well-Being Lifestyle

Keep up a healthy lifestyle that includes getting enough sleep, eating a balanced food, and exercising frequently. An immune system that is robust and in good condition is more capable of warding off diseases.

13. Appropriate Use of Antibiotics:

Only take antibiotics as directed by a medical practitioner, and make sure you finish the recommended course of treatment. Antibiotic resistance may be exacerbated by incomplete antibiotic courses.

14. Examining and removing colonialism:

Targeted decolonization procedures and Staph colonization screening may be taken into consideration in specific high-risk scenarios or healthcare environments.

Individuals with weakened immune systems, those with long-term medical illnesses, and those living in healthcare facilities or community housing should pay special attention to preventive measures. People can lower their risk of contracting Staph infections and improve community health by adopting these preventive measures into their daily lives.

If staph infections are not properly and quickly treated, they may cause problems and negatively affect a person's health in the long run. The type of infection, the strain of Staphylococcus bacteria involved, the body part affected, and the general health of the person all determine how serious the problems are. The following are some possible side effects and long-term effects of Staph infections:

1. Transmission of Infection:

If left untreated, Staph infections have the potential to spread to other body sites, resulting in more serious infections and consequences.

2. Formation of Abscesses:

Abscesses, or collections of pus inside tissues that may need to be drained, can develop as a result of Staph infections, particularly those that affect the skin and soft tissues.

3. Infections with the System:

Severe Staph infections can cause bloodstream infections (bacteremia), which can develop into sepsis a potentially fatal illness marked by extensive inflammation and organ failure.

4. Osteomyelitis:

Osteomyelitis, an infection of the bone, can result from Staph infections and can have long-term consequences, including damage to the bone.

5. Septic arthritis:

If treatment for septic arthritis is delayed or inadequate, it can lead to inflammation, joint damage, and reduced mobility.

6. Endocarditis:

An infection of the heart's inner lining and heart valves known as staphylococcal endocarditis can cause damage to the heart valves and long-term cardiac problems.

7. recurring infections

Recurrent infections may be more likely in those with a history of Staph infections, particularly those brought on by strains of the infection that are resistant to antibiotics, such as MRSA.

8. Prolonged Skin Disorders:

Changes in skin texture, scarring, and chronic skin disorders can all be attributed to severe or recurring skin infections.

9. Resistance to Antibiotics:

Antibiotic-resistant strains of Staph infections can arise as a result of prolonged or improper use of antibiotics, making treatment of subsequent infections more difficult.

10. Effect on Life Quality:

Severe or chronic Staph infections can seriously impair a person's quality of life by interfering with day-to-day activities, employment, and general wellbeing.

11. Associated infections with healthcare:

Staph infections in healthcare settings can result in longer hospital stays, more medical expenses, and more patient difficulties.

12. Complications Following Infection:

- Even after the infection has been treated, some people may continue to have post-infectious consequences, such as autoimmune reactions or persistent symptoms.

13. Transfer to Other Parties:

Staph infections can transfer resistant germs to others in community or clinical settings, especially if the strains are resistant to antibiotics.

Efficient diagnosis, suitable management, and compliance with prophylactic measures are essential in mitigating the difficulties and enduring consequences linked to Staph infections. People who exhibit symptoms that could indicate a Staph infection should get medical help right once, especially if they have underlying medical conditions. This will stop the illness from spreading and lower the chance of complications.

CONCLUSION

In summary, Staphylococcus bacteria, which cause Staph infections, can cause a variety of ailments, from minor skin infections to serious, life-threatening diseases. In healthcare and community settings, Staphylococcus aureus presents a serious threat due to its capacity to cause infections and acquire drug resistance, especially methicillin-resistant forms.

Effective management of Staph infections requires early diagnosis, proper antibiotic therapy, and prevention measures. Keeping oneself clean, taking care of wounds, and not sharing personal objects all help lower the chance of infection.

Staph infections can have serious long-term effects and complications, particularly if the infection is not treated or if antibiotic resistance grows. Among the possible outcomes include infection spread, abscess formation, systemic problems, and effects on quality of life.

Healthcare practitioners are essential in the management of infections, the responsible use of antibiotics, and the prompt and focused treatment of Staph infections. To improve results and stop resistant strains from spreading further, ongoing research and actions to combat antibiotic resistance are crucial.

People are advised to take precautions to protect themselves and others, including getting medical help as soon as they suspect they may have a Staph infection. People may help avoid and manage Staph infections by being aware of the hazards, maintaining proper hygiene, and working with healthcare professionals. This will ultimately improve people's general health and well-being.

THE END